I0415184

Street Workout

Lose Weight and Gain Muscle Mass with Highly Effective Street Exercises

Table of Contents

Introduction 5

What is Street Workout? 6

The Growing Phenomena of Calisthenics 7

So Who Should Partake in Street Workout? 8

How Calisthenics Can Transform Your Life 9

The Insane Benefits of the Street Exercises 9

A Boost in Your Endurance 10

Enhanced Muscle Flexibility 10

Dynamic Increase in Overall Strength 12

You Can Target Your Upper Body 12

You Can Target Your Lower Body 13

Calisthenics Help Burn a Heck Lot of Calories 14

How Can I Start Bodyweight Exercises? 15

Place Yourself into Encouraging and Motivating
Environment 16

Harness the Power of the Social Media 16

Do Not Ignore Your Body 17

Maintain a Proper Diet 17

Start From the Basics - Ignore Everybody Else 18

Stay Focused and Committed to the WORK 19

How to Get Your Nutrition Right 20

Superfoods to Include in Your Diet 21

Eggs 23

Include Flaxseeds into Your Diet 23

Berries 23

Oatmeal 25

Sweet Potatoes..26

Broccoli...26

Start Drinking Green Tea 27

Spinach 27

Dried Fruits and Nuts 28

Oranges...29

Yogurt 30

Altering your Lifestyle for Better Results.....................31

Drink Plenty of Water 31

Don't Forget to Keep Your Body Moving 32

Invest in Some Good Probiotics 32

Brisk Walk 33

Breathing 34

Retrain Your Brain 34

The Goals You Set Have to Be Achievable 35

Get an Encouraging Support System 36

Stick With a Routine...37

Street Workout Exercises: Entry-Level 39

Street Workout for Gaining Muscle Bulk & Strength 40

Pull-ups on the Horizontal Bar....................................40

Isometric Hold on the Pull-up Bar 41

Bench Dips..42

Leg Raises 44

Street Workout for Losing Weight................................45

Jumping Rope as a Workout...45

Buying the Right Jumping Rope...................................49

Advanced Level Street Workout Exercises....................51

Push-Ups...51

Push-Up on Bars 51

One-Arm Push-Ups 52

One Leg Squats AKA "The Gun" 54

Street Workouts for a Toned and Dream Body 56

The Human Flag 56

The Fro`nt Vis 56

The Importance of Rest and Recovery 58

Tips on How to Gain Muscle Mass 59

Never Stop Doing Resistance Training 59

Eat Your Proteins 59

Sleep Tight and Sleep Right 60

Carefully Increase your Weight 61

Rest and Recovery...61

The Importance of a Proper Sleep Cycle for Increased Muscle Repair 62

Conclusion...64

Introduction

Needless to say, when you hear the word 'workout,' first of all you think about the gym. Regardless of what most people think, there is more to working out than running on a treadmill, and that's what street workout is all about. But what is it anyway and how can it help you gain muscle mass? Well, that's precisely the kind of questions we'll be discussing in this eBook.

What is Street Workout?

There is no doubts that street workout has grown in popularity all over the world. The basis of every exercise in a street workout comes from one of the earliest forms of strength and agility training, known as 'calisthenics.' Street workout involves the use of your body weight to strengthen and tone your muscles. You would be surprised to know that Spartans, as well as various types of legendary warriors, relied on calisthenics to gain muscle mass and improve their strength. No wonder that warriors from earlier times had incredible strength, agility, flexibility, and endurance.

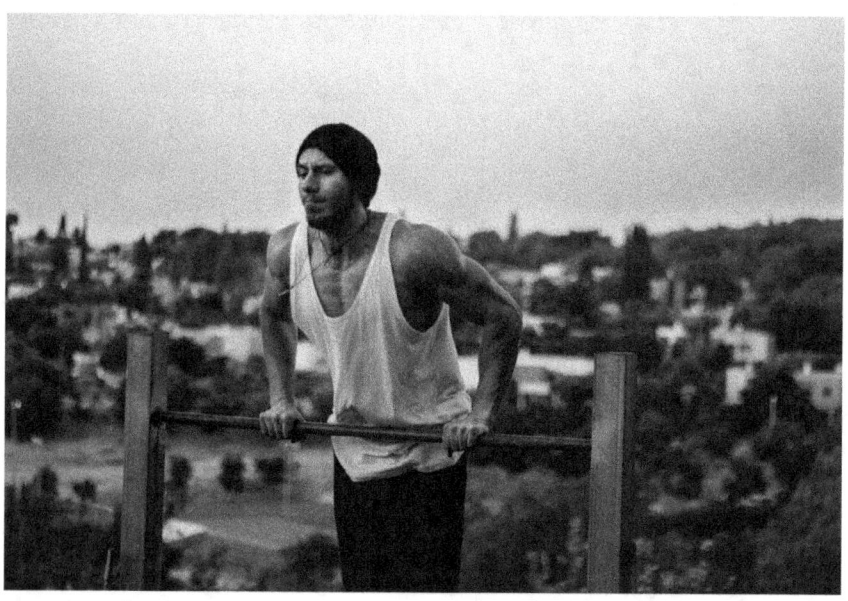

Today, calisthenics translates into street workout, which has become a buzzword in the fitness world. Moreover, basic calisthenics exercises are used by renowned gymnasts, and incorporated into training of military squads and Special Forces regiments. Not to mention that sportsmen such as tennis, football and basketball players also prefer calisthenic exercises.

The Growing Phenomena of Calisthenics

Street workout has turned into a modern terminology for bodyweight exercises that you can perform outdoors. You can think of it as a unique and barrier-free way of improving and enhancing your health and maintaining your body in perfect shape. Street workout incorporates an entirely new set of elements; it is creative in its own right, the exercises can be improvised to match your strength and flexibility levels, it promotes a healthier way of living and can be considered an entirely new type of sport.

This type of workout appeals to individuals with different walks of life. Regardless of your starting point or the fact that you've been living an inactive life for a long time, it doesn't take much to start a street workout regimen.

One of the most notable facts about calisthenics is that the workouts are extremely versatile. You can use many different exercises and techniques of using your bodyweight to burn calories, improve muscle mass and gain strength. Street workout exercises are not exclusive for any one type of sport, which is why so many schools encourage kids to perform these exercises in their PE classes.

In addition, street workout is universal in the sense that it is not gender-specific; it has no age restrictions; the accessibility of this workout methodology is what has made it so popular today.

So Who Should Partake in Street Workout?

The undeniable fact is that as we age, our muscle mass gradually decline. The scientific term for this is sarcopenia. Muscle mass usually begins to decrease in people within the age brackets of 30 to 80. They will experience a loss of 30% to 50% of total muscle strength - and as you have guessed, this will prove to be one of the biggest hindrances in maintaining an active and healthy lifestyle as gaining more energy will become difficult. However, inactive lifestyle will only aggravate this process of losing muscle mass.

Despite the adverse effects of loss of muscle mass, people in their mid-thirties, forties or above will start to feel more hesitant and reluctant to try and enhance their strength and level of fitness through a combination of resistance exercises. Most people falsely believe that if they've lived an inactive life, there is no way they can just start exercising at a later stage. You have to understand that it is never too late to start working out. All you need is determination, a healthy diet, and the right mindset. With these elements, you can't fail to improve your body tone, enhance your strength, and quite possibly you can gain more muscle bulk.

How Calisthenics Can Transform Your Life

So why should you move over to calisthenics anyway? In this section, we'll be discussing the unbelievable benefits of calisthenics.

The Insane Benefits of the Street Exercises

One of the reasons why calisthenics have become widely accepted form of keeping fit is the fact that these training methods are attractive for all sorts of people. The training is easy, and you will never need any type of equipment to tone your body. In light of this, some exciting reasons are mentioned below why calisthenics will completely transform your life.

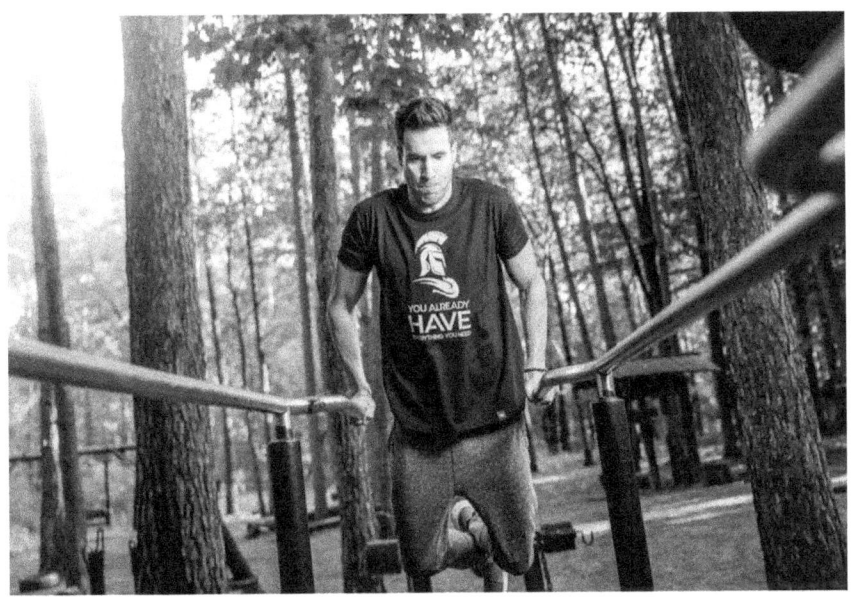

A Boost in Your Endurance

Using calisthenic exercises in the form of circuit training is a pretty intense way of developing muscle endurance. If you perform multiple activities repeatedly, three to four sets in about 15 minutes with 10 to 15 seconds of rest between sets; your body will start to build resistance to daily exhaustion and fatigue. You think of this circuit training as, some would suggest, a better alternative to traditional cardiovascular exercises such as high-intensity interval training on the treadmill or the elliptical machine.

If you dedicate yourself to training and perform the exercises every other day, your body will start getting stronger and stronger each day, making it easier for you to push yourself further and perform more repetitions and sets before exhausting your muscles.

Enhanced Muscle Flexibility

Most exercises that constitute a street workout require a certain level of flexibility from your muscles and body. For instance, lunges actively involve your hip muscles allowing you to stretch your legs while keeping one leg behind you. The movement needs fluid flexibility for smoother repetitions. In addition, you might experience different muscular restrictions while performing this exercise if you haven't done it for a long time. That is precisely why using your own weight to stretch your leg muscles via calisthenic techniques will identify where you lack in flexibility. Pushing yourself a bit further every day will improve your flexibility, allowing you to perform more reps and sets.

By increasing strength and flexibility constantly, your body will quickly adapt to this change in flexibility levels, making it easier for you to perform every exercise like a professional. In addition, calisthenics enables you to increase your overall range of motion, which in turn allows your body to incorporate the use of all the right muscle groups to perform different exercises. However, it is essential that you perform all the necessary stretching movements prior to targeting any single body part. If you're doing a leg workout, first give them a good stretch to make the joints and muscles more fluid and to encourage a proper range of motion.

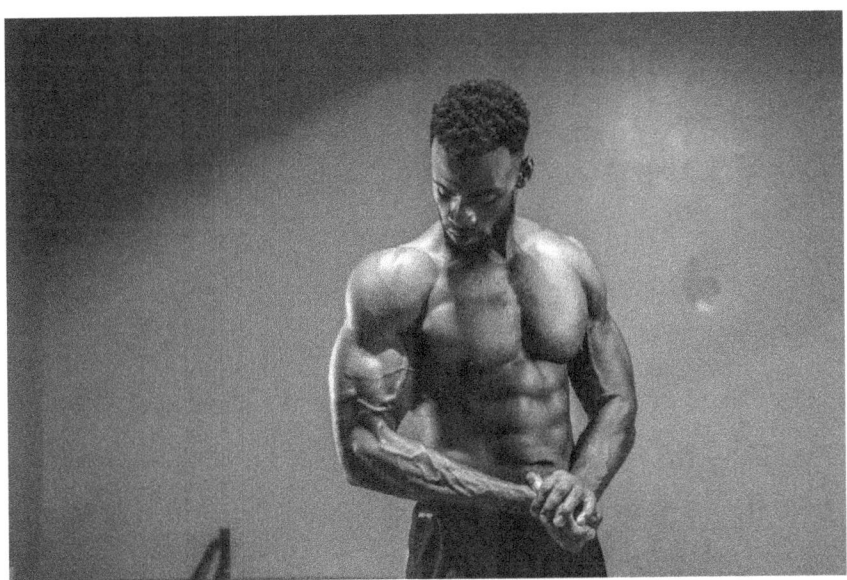

Dynamic Increase in Overall Strength

There's no doubt that street workout will help build your overall strength and improve your muscle mass and growth. However, what most people don't know is that it doesn't just enhance your muscles — calisthenics or bodyweight exercises also promote bone and joint health. Calisthenic exercises are widely used in US Army training at a very basic level. Beyond helping you build muscle strength, this type of training also dramatically decreases any chance of injury. Moreover, if you've never opted for weight training because of the impact it has on your joints and the fact that it gives you stretch marks, a street workout is perfect for you because bodyweight exercises do not come with the usual wear and tear that other forms of exercises do.

You Can Target Your Upper Body

One of the best advantages of street workout is the fact that you can incorporate a variety of different exercises to target your whole upper body. Some popular exercises include pull-ups and push-ups. These are some of the fundamental exercises you can practice to build incredible muscle strength and tone up your body. You can employ both these popular exercises in different techniques when you are performing circuit training. Push-ups target your chest, develop all three tricep heads, develop your shoulders and build your core.

Pull-ups, on the other hand, target your lower and upper-back muscles, shoulders and biceps.

You can start with performing different variants of both exercises. For example, when it comes to push-ups, you can perform clap push-ups, diamond push-ups, shoulder taps, etc. With pull-up, you can use the wide grip or the narrow grip to target different areas of the back. Moreover, using the under grip, you can build bicep strength and mass. Pull-ups also enhance your grip strength.

You Can Target Your Lower Body

Just as pull-ups are great for building your upper and lower back, squatting exercises are good for building muscles of your lower body. However, prior to doing any leg exercise it is essential to ensure that there is a lot of activation in your hip muscles, specifically your glutes.

The best way to fire your glutes is to perform short sets of bridges. Moreover, if you are new to squatting or haven't performed this exercise for a long time, never push yourself over the edges of your ability and range of motion when you're squatting or doing lunges. There are a slew of different variations when it comes to squatting. You can choose exercises that suit your level of flexibility at the time, adding new exercises gradually and increasing number of repetitions. For example, you can begin with the standard arms-crossed-at-front squatting. Also, you can perform seated leg extensions.

Calisthenics Help Burn a Heck Lot of Calories

Another reason why calisthenics is more beneficial in terms of overall fitness is the fact that the exercises combine a mixture of cardio and resistance training. These exercises enable you to perform both aerobic and anaerobic movements. Exercises with these two elements, for example, power jump, burpees, and bear crawl incorporate the use of your total body weight, building muscle while also burning calories, i.e. excess fat.

Moreover, the fact that street workout exercises make you alter your body position constantly, yet consistently, will allow you to maintain a high heart rate while building strength.

How Can I Start Bodyweight Exercises?

Starting calisthenic exercises is easy - all you need to do is start from the basics, which is combining some popular exercises to gain strength and stamina. Exercises like push-ups, pull-ups, tricep dips, etc. are all popular exercises that you can perform almost anywhere without need for extensive equipment. Moreover, these exercises also provide a high rate of regression with every movement. For people who do not know what regression is - it is a simpler and more basic movement of an exercise or movement. What it basically does is gradually make it easier for you to perform advanced levels of movements for each exercise, getting rid of any muscular restrictions you could have experienced when you started these exercises. You get stronger with each day of training!

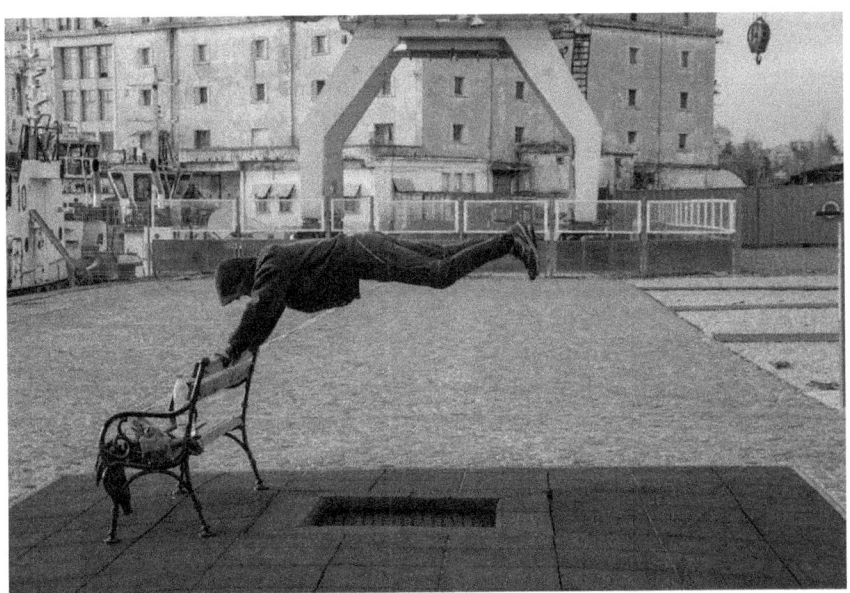

In light of this, here are some very invigorating and important factors you must incorporate in your everyday life to get stronger, leaner and fitter no matter who you are and how old you are.

Place Yourself into Encouraging and Motivating Environment

If you dwell amongst people who constantly bicker about how life has battered them down or how it is impossible to make lifestyle changes at a certain age, the chances are high that you give up before you even start.

Starting your journey to a more active lifestyle becomes much easier when you surround yourself with people and peers that are a constant source of confidence and motivation. Meet with 'can-do' people, go online and listen to how people have transformed their bodies, go out with friends who will always push you to achieve a bit more - not just in your workouts, but in your life as well. Positive mindset is paramount to healthy mind and body!

Harness the Power of the Social Media

Social media can become an overwhelming source of doubt, or it can be one of the most motivating things in the world. However, you must not let social media intimidate you from transforming your life. Sure, you will come across a slew of videos where the skill and talent and fitness levels of trainers and other people will absolutely knock you off the wall. But you cannot afford to be disappointed or feel pessimistic about achieving those fitness levels. Do not compare yourself with other people, you are who you are and only 'you' can motivate yourself to make real what seemed to be impossible.

Do Not Ignore Your Body

You have to understand that when you start calisthenic exercises, your body will naturally feel fatigued and you will experience muscle exhaustion. But this is totally normal! There will inevitably be muscle soreness when you're performing multiple sets and different exercises every day. However, it is also vital to distinguish between pains that result from working out and the pain you may experience as a result of a possible injury.

Stay determined to develop a strong base while performing exercises and muscle movements exactly the way they are meant to be performed. This will drastically reduce the chances of any injuries and increase your chances of efficiently building more muscle mass. As you progress, your body will gradually begin to tell you when you're pushing yourself too far and when it's time to ease up.

Maintain a Proper Diet

One of the major factors in developing a healthy body is the fuel you put into it. If you're really determined to build a leaner and healthier body, you have to be serious about quitting foods that adversely affect your health. Stop eating processed foods, sugary snacks and things that have an empty calorie count. Learn how to include healthy alternatives to your usual diet to get the best nutrition possible. For optimal performance and desirable results, you need to watch what you eat.

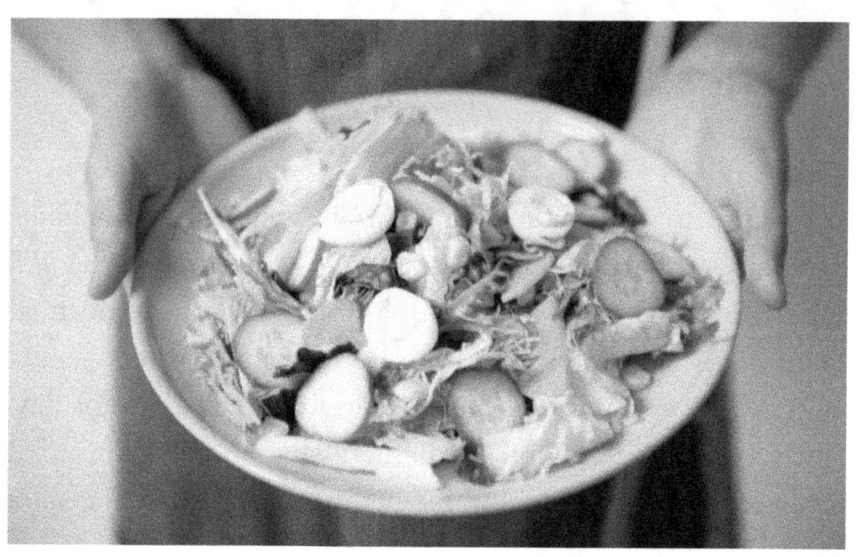

Start From the Basics - Ignore Everybody Else

If you have never lifted weight or performed any sort of exercises in your life, the way you start and progress will be different from the way of an individual in a good physical condition. No matter what you do, don't compare your fitness level or strength with someone with an athletic background. You will have to start from the basics and build your strength and muscle mass from scratch. It doesn't matter if you can't do a single pull-up; try doing an assisted repetition instead of pushing yourself from the first day, the same applied from the different combination of exercises you perform. Slow and steady wins the race.

It is immensely important for you to motivate yourself and maintain your commitment to active lifestyle. You must remain determined to get better each day. And as you progress, as you get stronger and more flexible, you will automatically start to incorporate different variations of the exercises you perform. But for now, do everything in a step-by-step manner - do not try to achieve everything at once.

It is never too late to finally get into shape. Sure, your progress and fitness journey will not be the same as shape and progress of any other person, but it is worth knowing that it is your own journey - enjoy every moment of it, celebrate your progress, record your gains, count your calories; living an active lifestyle is really a very fun and rewarding thing to do - and the best part of it is that this is a lifelong commitment.

Stay Focused and Committed to the WORK

If you want to see effective results of your workouts, it is important to always remain focused on the quality of the exercises you perform. Quality dictates the amount of muscle strength and flexibility that you will gain. That is why it is important that no matter how long you train for or how many exercises you perform, working harder, smarter and with increased consistency will help you gain more muscle mass and strength over time.

Do not become frustrated if you see that your progress comes slowly every day. The important thing is to remember everything you do correctly will keep adding on and accumulating gradually into something bigger.

How to Get Your Nutrition Right

It is utterly essential to learn the importance of nutrition, as it is the only way to fuel your progress and to lead to a fitter and healthier lifestyle. Eating the right foods promotes your overall health, but they also act as solid bedrock for your attempts to enhance your muscle tone and keep your body clean. You have to select a variety of clean foods that are rich in necessary nutrients, vitamins, proteins, healthy fats, and carbohydrates to make your transformation smooth and effective.

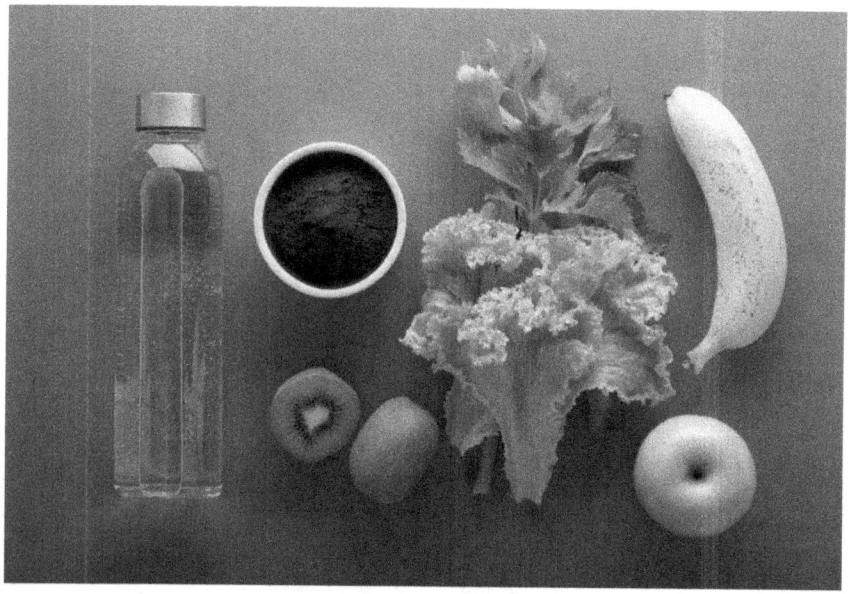

Dietary proteins sources such as grilled chicken, boiled beef, and boiled eggs, are good sources of vital amino acids for making new muscle tissue after your workout. Dietary carbohydrates are sources of energy that will help maintain your muscle stamina, providing you with the strength you need every day. These carbohydrates also play an instrumental role in restoring your body's energy stores through the production of glycogen.

Dietary fats account for about 70% of your body's total energy supply when you're resting. These fats also promote healthy metabolism and naturally propel the production of various vitamins such as vitamins D, K, A and E. Furthermore, these vitamins help maintain the necessary amount of testosterone required to keep on building new muscle tissue and mass.

These are all important nutrients that you will need on a daily basis to help get closer and closer to your fitness goals. And when you talk about a clean diet, you cannot omit any one of these nutrient types. You have to incorporate all three types into your diet.

The best thing about these nutrients is that you can get them from eating regular things such as fruits, vegetables, meat, dairy products, etc. The accessibility factor of these nutrients is what makes clean eating affordable and highly effective.

Superfoods to Include in Your Diet

Superfoods are pretty prominent when you talk about healthy eating and fitness. These are some of the best types of foods you can incorporate into your everyday diet. Superfoods can supplement your overall health in addition to the healthy food you eat. They contain a plethora of nutrients, amino acids, antioxidants and disease-combating elements that everybody should get with their food.

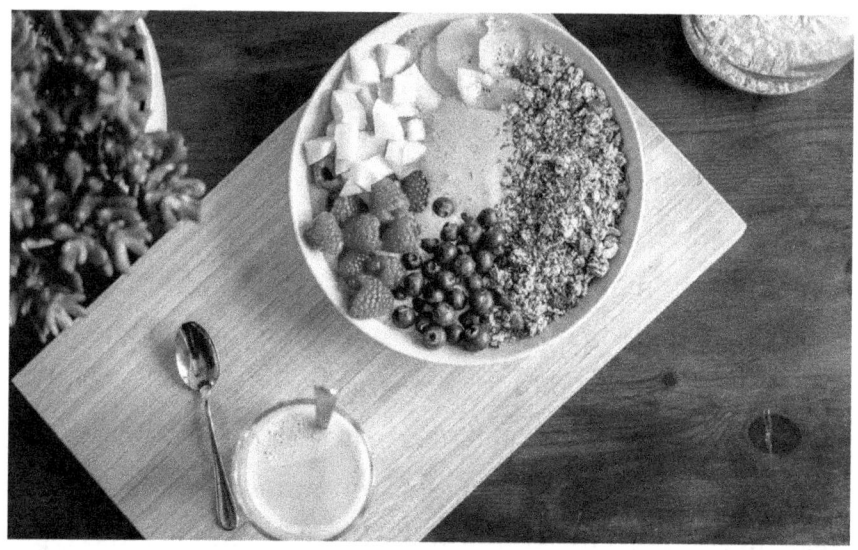

It is also important to understand that some products that come into the superfood category can be really expensive and impossible to incorporate into your daily diet. That is why it is essential to stick to foods that are easily accessible and do not put a heavy burden on your budget. You don't have to go for something rare and expensive, like sardines or goji berries, to build up your muscles and boost your fitness. There is a whole range of superfoods that can appear in your fridge quickly and without extra expenses.

So without further adieu, here are some of the best superfoods you can eat to maintain a strong and healthy body:

Eggs

Eggs are rich in amino acids and are packed with easily digestible protein. A single egg contains about 70 calories. By eating one egg, you get 6 grams of high-quality protein. Moreover, egg yolks contain two very powerful antioxidants (zeaxanthin and lutein). Both these antioxidants help to maintain health of your eyes.

In fact, people who eat whole eggs or about 18 grams of protein, which is three eggs, after intense resistance training, show a lot of muscle growth through a natural process known as protein synthesis.

Include Flaxseeds into Your Diet

If you want to speed up results, there is nothing better you can do than to start eating flaxseeds as a snack. Along with being low on the calorie count, flaxseeds increase your fiber intake, keeping you fuller for longer. Also, flaxseeds are rich in different types of vital minerals and nutrients, particularly in omega-3 fatty acids, which also help eliminate any symptoms of obesity while keeping your slim. And, according to various sources, flaxseeds also tame your appetite, which means you won't have those hunger pangs.

Berries

Berries, such as strawberries, blueberries or blackberries, contain large amounts of natural fiber. Fiber is a staple nutrient that is responsible for keeping your metabolism clean and running. Moreover, it is also great for your heart as it flushes out all the bad cholesterol from your body, cleaning the arteries and promoting your cardiovascular health.

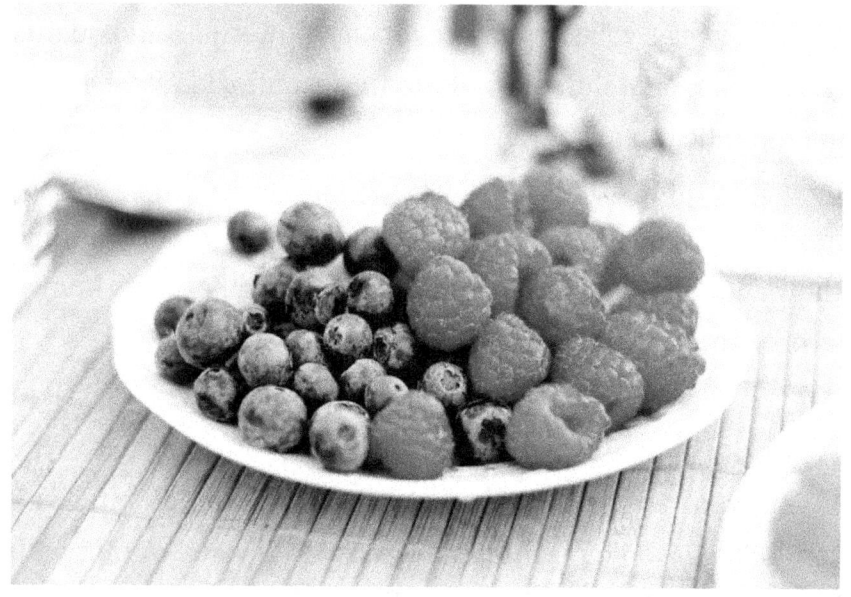

In fact, you don't need to have each and every type of berries; you can eat strawberries and blueberries if they are easily accessible. But perhaps the best part about berries is the fact that they can be incorporated into a number of different types of meals. If you don't like eating a plain old bowl of oatmeal, try slicing a couple of strawberries or blueberries and just garnish your oatmeal with it, and you have a delicious meal. You can also prepare smoothies using raspberries; this will provide you with lots of fiber, so if you're on a diet, it's a good addition to your menu. While strawberries contain vitamin C and a fiber count of 3 grams per cup, blueberries contain 4 grams of fiber per cup and contain antioxidants and anthocyanins.

Oatmeal

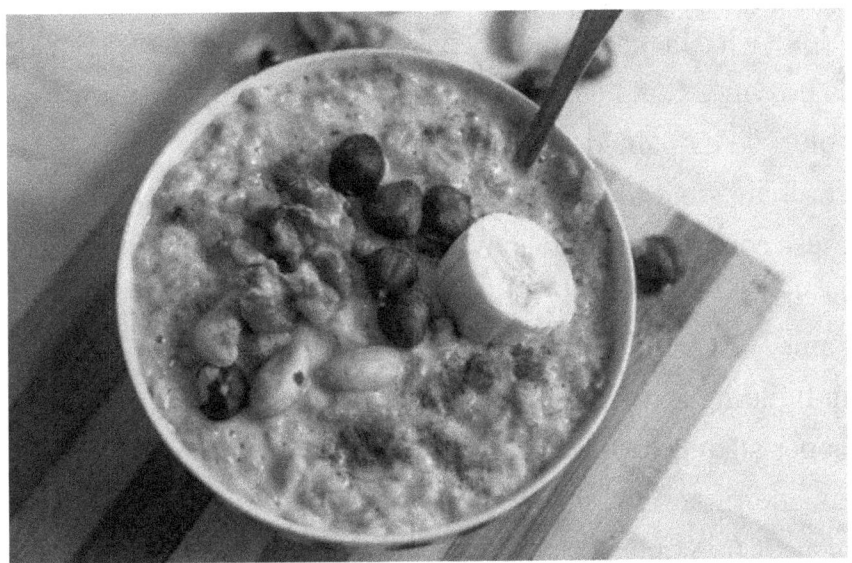

Oatmeal is an incredible breakfast meal and a staple in many countries. Oats supply your body with fiber, which is an important health factor that many people are deficient in. To get rid of all that bad cholesterol that may clog up your veins and lead to several cardiovascular problems, your stomach needs fiber to flush it all out of the system. This also makes oatmeal a perfect calisthenic workout meal to boost your metabolism and

keep the blood flowing to your heart, gradually increasing your stamina. Moreover, plain oats do not contain any natural or unnatural sugar. To make oatmeal even healthier, you can add other superfoods such as blueberries, bananas, strawberries, kiwis or dried fruits and nuts to take your health up a notch.

Sweet Potatoes

Along with being absolutely delicious, sweet potatoes are rich in enzymes that help keep the body functioning. Their orange color is explained by large amounts of beta and alpha-carotene stored in sweet potatoes. Your body quickly absorbs these components and converts them into vitamin A, which is necessary for keeping your immune system at the top of its game. Not to mention, vitamin A also plays a supporting role in building muscle tissue, ensures eye health and keeps your bones stronger for longer time.

In addition, the phytochemicals form a protective barrier against free radicals, eliminating them before they turn into a serious health risk for you. Half a cup of sweet potatoes contains various nutrients such as zeaxanthin, lutein, vitamin C, potassium, and vitamin B6.

Broccoli

You may not necessarily like broccoli, but the vegetable is packed with a powerhouse of nutrients that promote bone health. Broccoli contains three types of vitamins, namely A, C, and K, all of which help to keep your bones healthy. Broccoli also contains folates. Another reason why broccoli is on the top of the list of superfoods is the fact that it contains a cancer-fighting component called sulforaphane. This component fights free radicals and protects enzymes of the body from impact of toxins.

Start Drinking Green Tea

Green tea is a wonderful thing, packed with catechins; the enzymes boost your metabolism, optimizing the level of fat you can burn. Green tea is also good at expelling unnecessary water from your body, since it is a diuretic. In addition, the hot beverage also decreases your body's capability to absorb fat. Drink about 2 to 3 cups every day along with performing exercises to look trim and slim.

Spinach

Leafy greens add a whole lot of minerals and vitamins and a generous amount of disease-fighting enzymes, keeping your body clean and detoxified, along with aiding to boost muscle growth and stamina. Spinach, in particular, is an abundant source of vitamins K, C, and A. Moreover, the dark leafy green vegetable contains minerals, such as magnesium and potassium, as well as vitamin E, fiber, and calcium. Apart from keeping your body fit, spinach can also help with your weight loss efforts, keeping the mind fresh. And also, according to scientific research data, the leafy green can also help fight free radicals, thus helping to prevent and combat cancer.

Dried Fruits and Nuts

Dried fruits and nuts are nature's healthiest snacks. Enriched with all sorts of polyunsaturated fats along with a healthy dose of magnesium, (both of which are vital for health of your cardiovascular system), nuts like almonds will become a shield against multiple health complications such as insulin resistance, which may lead to the development of symptoms associated with Type-2 diabetes.

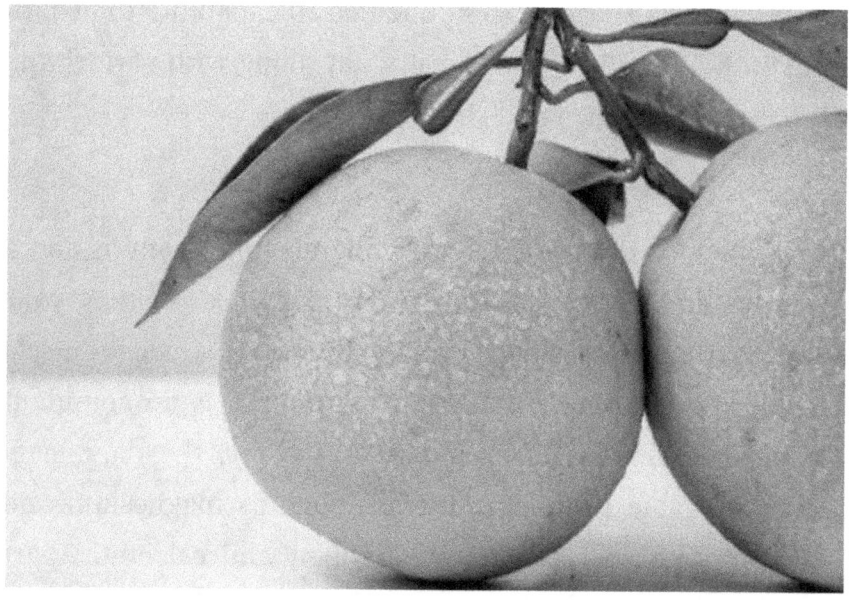

Nuts also contain antioxidants such as resveratrol and ellagic, both of which massively help to protect your body against the devastating effects of free radicals, which may lead to cancer.

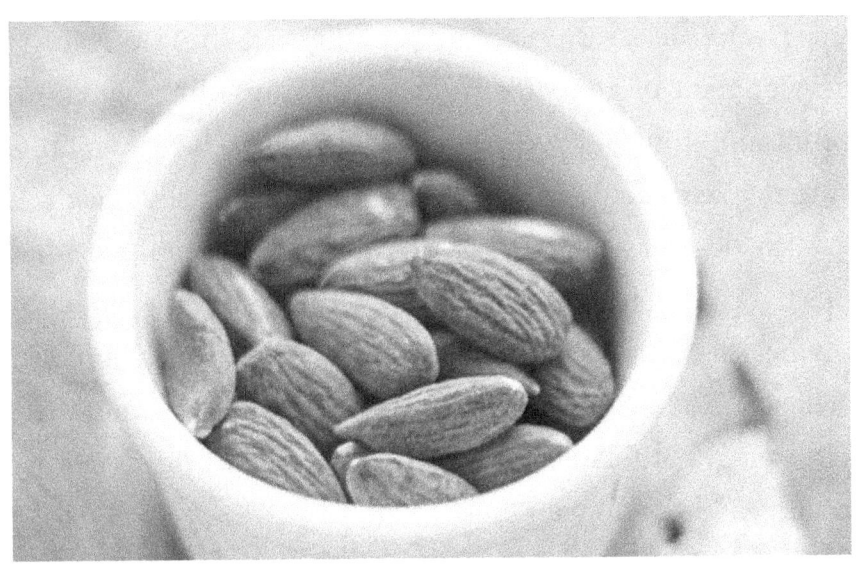

In addition, dried fruits and nuts will also provide your body with generous quantities of fiber. According to multiple studies, fiber is a key element in keeping the bad bacteria in your gut at bay - boosting your bowel movement and eliminating any symptoms of constipation. You can incorporate nuts in your diet in multiple ways if you don't want to eat them whole, you can get organic nut butter and eat it with bread, or you can even blend them with low-fat milk and drink the mixture as a supplement.

Oranges

Nowadays many people are skeptical about the power of oranges. However, the fruit is a valuable source of multiple nutrients, as well as a healthy natural storage of vitamin C; and vitamin C is a vital nutrient that helps keeping the body free from diseases, plays important role in the natural development of antibodies, and keeps your white blood cell count up, thus taking part in maintaining your immune system clean and strong. Moreover, your body needs a healthy dose of vitamin C to fight off infections and maladies like the common cold or flu at bay. Oranges are also good for the health of your skin, the enzymes in the fruit help boost collagen production in order to keep your skin nice and firm. With plenty of folates and some fiber, oranges can be a very healthy addition to your diet.

Yogurt

When it comes to gut health and a clean metabolism, yogurt is one of the most beneficial dietary foods you can get. This superfood is full of probiotics necessary to keep your metabolism boosted. Moreover, yogurt is an excellent source of calcium, along with other vital nutrients and minerals such as vitamin B12, phosphorus, zinc, potassium, protein, and riboflavin. For muscle tone and development, it is recommended that you go for Greek yogurt to gain muscle bulk more effectively and in a more healthy way. For added benefits, it is also wise if you choose plain yogurt instead of flavored ones as they contain artificial sweeteners.

Altering your Lifestyle for Better Results

So let's say that you already eat healthy foods and greens, and perform plenty of resistance exercises, is there really any need to get your lifestyle in check beyond that? Well, the answer is yes! Although healthy eating is a big part of maintaining your physical fitness, there are still numerous factors that may inhibit proper muscle growth, strength, and stamina.

Moreover, in all honesty, healthy eating is a complex challenge. You have to choose wisely what you eat, which is why there are several tweaks that you can make in your lifestyle to keep the fitness cycle going no matter what. These factors will not only physically benefit you but may help prolong your life for a couple of years and make you a very happy individual in the later periods of your life.

In light of this, below are mentioned some very important factors that you should consider:

Drink Plenty of Water

Dehydration is a big no-no when it comes to practically anything - especially when performing resistance training. In addition, 70% of your body is water, which means adequate hydration contributes to muscle mass and tone. Without the sufficient amount of water in your body you will achieve nothing, no matter how healthy you eat or how regularly you exercise. Instead, you will start feeling exhausted even before you begin any exercise. Ideally, you must drink at least eight glasses of water throughout the day to harness more energy.

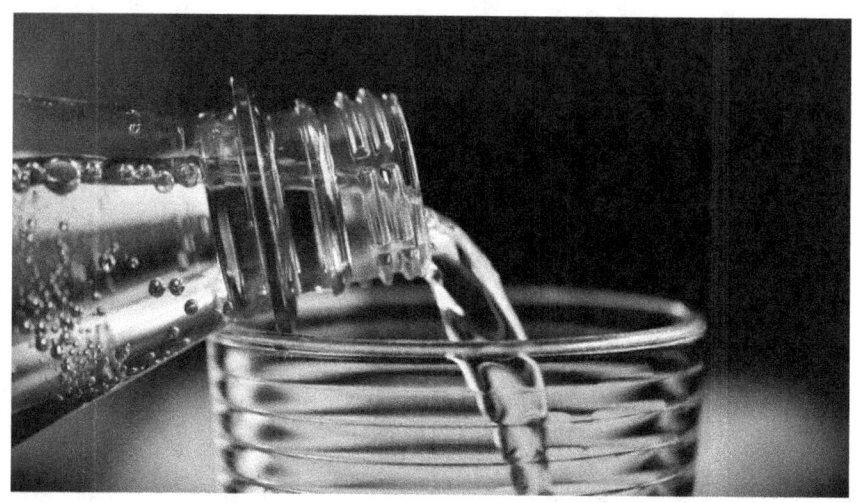

Don't Forget to Keep Your Body Moving

Surely, it is good that you perform calisthenics on the daily basis; however, even exercise will not be able to correct some of the problems that arise from sitting 6 to 8 hours a day hunched in front of your computer. You have to keep your body moving. Stand up and do stretches after every 20-30 minutes in your office. Climb a flight of stairs and back, keep the blood circulating. In fact, according to discoveries from recent scientific study, lot of advantages that come from exercise were completely eliminated in individuals who sit for long periods of time.

Invest in Some Good Probiotics

Selecting the right dietary supplement is a complicated task. However, thanks to breakthroughs in scientific research, medical professionals emphasize about how a clean and active gut can fight diseases and boost your overall health. Not to mention, a healthy gut promotes better mood and helps maintain your immune system strong, sensitive, and reactive. So make it your goal to invest in the best probiotics you can find.

Brisk Walk

Effort you put into performing calisthenics will undoubtedly grant you the results you wish to achieve; however there could be days when you don't really feel like working out at all. Instead of wasting the day in inactivity or snacking, it is better just to get up and walk around your neighborhood. You don't have to do this for the whole day, walking once or twice a day will help build your leg muscles and boost your stamina.

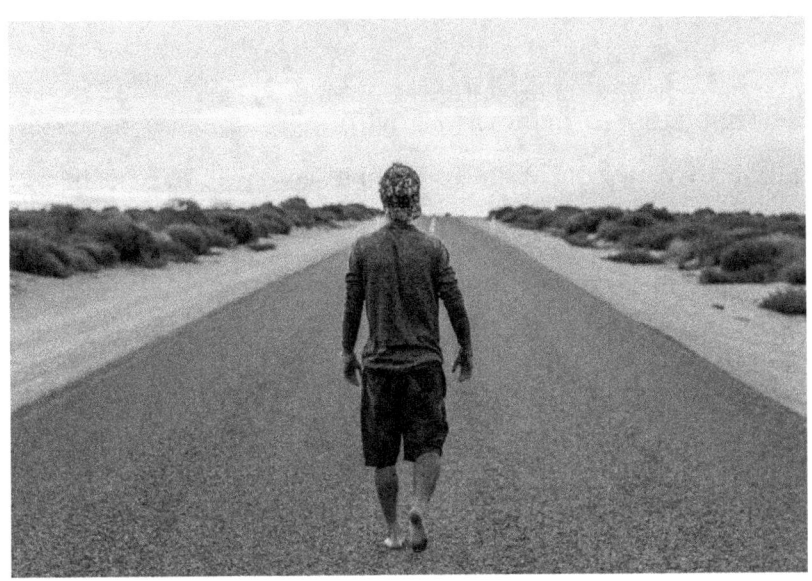

Breathing

Stress and anxiety have become a part of everybody's life. The daily routine of traveling from home to work and back home, balancing relationships, keeping up with friends, trying to stay fit and healthy — all this can take a heavy toll on the mind. Resisting stress has become hard in today's world. However, there are ways to stay positive and stress-free, and this is something that you do naturally anyway: breathing. The kind of breathing we're talking about has to be more focused and intended to relax your nerves. After you wake up in the morning, sit up straight in your bed without doing anything else, just for 5 to 8 minutes, take deep breaths from the stomach and exhale, close your eyes and envision yourself in a state of control, expelling all the negativity. Focused breathing is a hidden key to a calm mind and a healthy body.

Retrain Your Brain

The first step to achieving anything or making a massive change to your routine is to change your mind. You have to realize that only you possess the power to change yourself and your life for the better. But first you have to alter your mindset. Reset and re-evaluate. You have the ability to create multiple paths to success. However, the biggest obstacle you could ever face is the compulsion to distrust yourself, and once you overcome this, you can achieve anything you set out for, including building a healthier body and living a longer and healthier life.

You have to get real, pay close attention to all the things in your life affecting your emotions and behaviors, to understand how they influence you. Observe your life and ask yourself, are there any destructive habits causing problems in your life, like binge eating or self-loathing? Give yourself a pep talk in front of the mirror, say to yourself that you are going to make changes from now on; positive affirmation and focused self-visualization can help you boost your confidence, enhance your self-esteem, and propel you closer to your milestone with each passing day.

The Goals You Set Have to Be Achievable

You have to get real with the program. Have you ever envisioned the ultimate you? Contemplate on everything, narrow everything down and then put it into writing. Working out and building a healthier mind and body are quite serious milestones no different from achieving success at your work or personal life. You have to come up with both short- and long-term plans and milestones that you know you will be able to achieve, step by step.

Regardless of whether you're adding a new exercise to your street workout regimen, mastering a difficult exercise, checking your weight every week or learning how to prepare healthier foods or incorporate healthier nutrition habits, it is vital to set realistic and achievable life goals so that you can observe and record the changes to your body.

It is essential to remember to reward yourself for the efforts you have put in, but in a more life-affirming way - which essentially means, if you've hit a milestone; let's just say you've begun to notice the shredding on your abdominal muscles, creating an outline for your six packs - DO NOT reward yourself by eating a large pizza or a tasty, juicy cheeseburger. Treat yourself with a nice t-shirt instead!

Get an Encouraging Support System

It is important to understand that only you, and nobody else in the world, are responsible for driving your life to success. However, there are certain factors that help us get to where we want to be. A supportive family, good coworkers and best friends are also vital factors that sculpt you into the person you want to be and help achieve the objectives you wish to accomplish. You're more likely will get better results if you surround yourself with a healthy support system. It does not hurt to share your milestones with your family or friends. Talk to them about what you are doing to become fitter, discuss what you eat and take advice on how to incorporate even healthier habits in your life. Discuss your new street workout regimen with them.

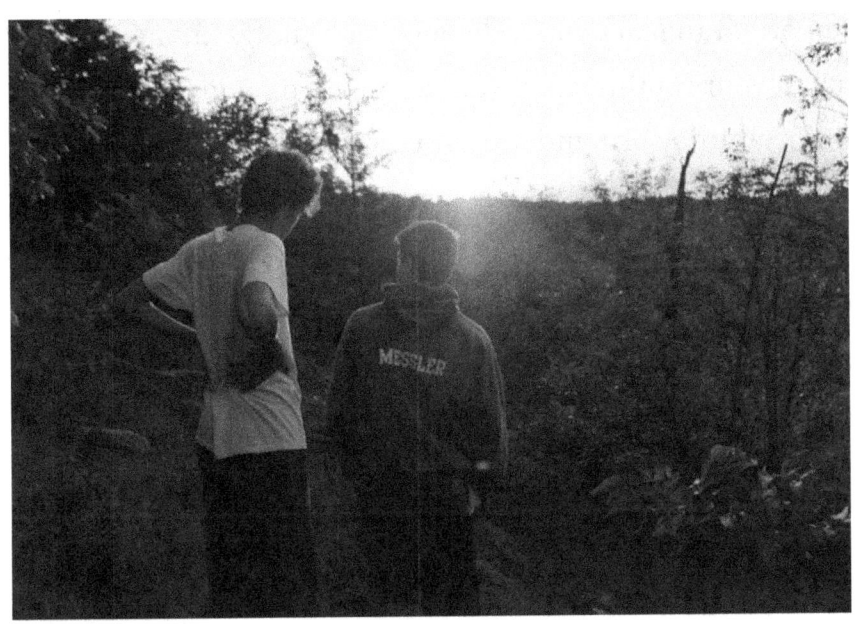

Moreover, if you're a smoker or if you drink a bit more than usual, talk to your friends, coworkers, and friends on how you can effectively cut back on these habits. You have to make them understand that getting healthy and fitter has become the central focus in your life and that their support has been previously and continues to be vital to you. Who knows, maybe you may just as well compel people to join you in your journey to become leaner and muscular.

Stick With a Routine

Once you started your journey to master calisthenics, making gains, looking leaner and stronger, at some point it can become difficult to stick with the routine. That is why it is important to mark your schedule, make notes on the calendar about your routine, what you're supposed to do from Monday onto Saturday or Sunday, set out a rest day in between, work through your important engagements throughout the day and set out time for your workout. With a good mindset, confidence and some self-assurance, you will be able to switch between your work and personal life, and never miss a day of workout as well.

Street Workout Exercises: Entry-Level

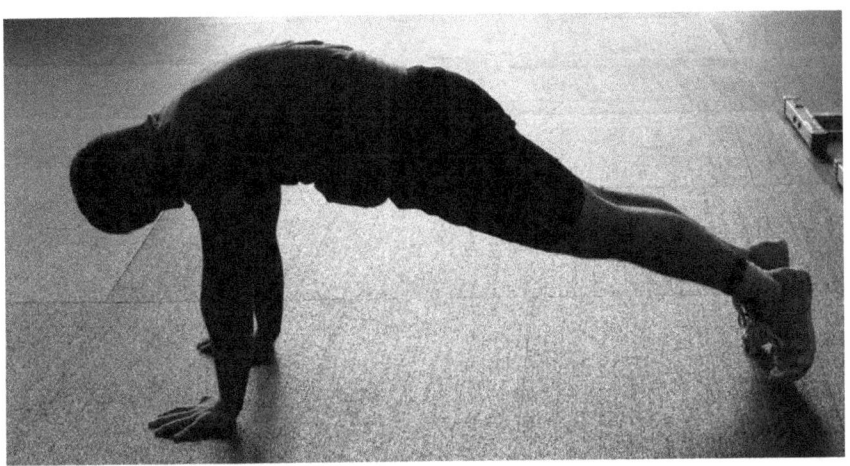

When it comes to calisthenics and muscle bulk gain, it is important to create a good workout routine and then to follow it closely. However, based on your levels of flexibility and strength you can quickly add more sophistication and repetition in your workout regimen. But it is also vital that you stick to exercises that are in alignment with objectives you are striving to accomplish. Calisthenics is for people of all shapes and sizes because you need little to no equipment at all. That also means that there is no 'one-size-fits-all' strategy in street workout. Fortunately, we have outlined a detailed set of calisthenic exercises you can start with, and then you can gradually take things up a notch with every passing month or week based on your level of fitness.

Street Workout for Gaining Muscle Bulk & Strength

Pull-ups on the Horizontal Bar

Pull-ups have become a widely neglected exercise because many see this exercise as overwhelming; you need to have a lot of arm strength to lift up your entire body weight. However, what many fail to understand is that doing pull-ups does not necessarily means you have to complete a set of 10 reps from the get-go. Professional bodybuilders say that even if you can do just one single pull-up, do it, then rest for 20-30 seconds and perform a second one. Gradually you will begin to see a massive improvement in your form and strength.

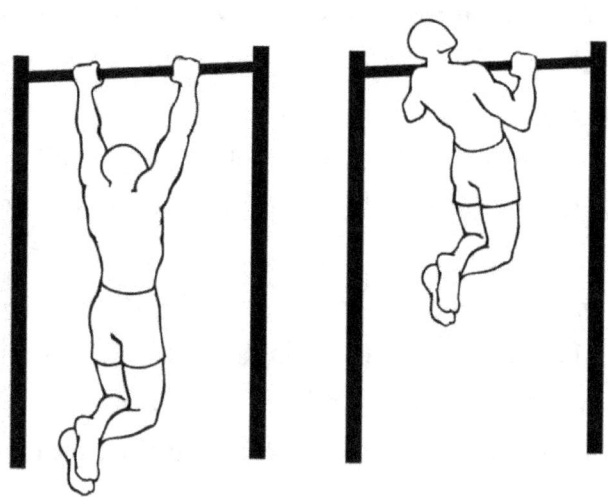

Pull-ups are a bare necessity when it comes to performing any kind of workout. Plus, this the best exercise to target your upper back, your traps, your chest and your shoulders. It is a complete workout methodology for muscle building, toning, and increasing your stamina. Moreover, it is also a good test to see your level of fitness if you're starting calisthenics after a long period of inactivity.

Pull-ups lay a foundation of your physical development. And there is no question that the exercise will keep on adding muscle mass on your biceps, your forearms, the rhomboid, and your lats. Assuming that you don't have a very bad level of fitness, it is safe to say that you might be able to perform about 2-4 pull-ups with your own weight. But if you have been training for a while and still do not have the strength to go beyond 8 to 10 reps, you need to reconsider your training and focus on increasing your strength, which means adding more protein and strength building foods in your diet.

Isometric Hold on the Pull-up Bar

It is important to start with the isometric technique because mastering this move will help you improve other forms of pull-ups. With a shoulder width grip on the pull-up bar, pull yourself up, bringing your chest in-line with the crossbar. Hold the position for about 10 or 15 seconds. Try to hold your shoulders as flat as you physically can and make sure that your chest is sticking out and forward.

After a couple of minutes of doing this, you will start to feel a burning sensation in the muscles of your upper back. These muscles are of utmost importance to perform more and more

41

pull-ups. No matter the intensity of the burn in your back muscles, keep on holding the position and tighten your back muscles.

Using isometric techniques is optimal for first-time calisthenic enthusiasts or people who have been inactive for a long time because if you do this exercise correctly, it will gradually target the muscles important for doing pull-ups the right way. And you will also gain more stamina and muscle mass over a longer period of training. But if you don't have enough strength to hold on, you can relax the shoulder blades after you feel the need to give up and shift the entire load on your forearms, biceps, and triceps.

It is recommended that you perform isometric holds with a straight grip in order to allocate maximum load on your upper back muscle. Grasping the pull-up bar with the reverse grip or with palms underneath the bar will increase load on your biceps.

Bench Dips

This is a mid-level exercise that utilizes body weight to tone your triceps. Since this exercise is fairly easy, it's perfect for beginners who are just entering the world of bodyweight training. However, it's worth mentioning that this particular exercise can be hard on your shoulders so if you've had a history of shoulder pain, you ought to consult your doctor before doing any bench dips.

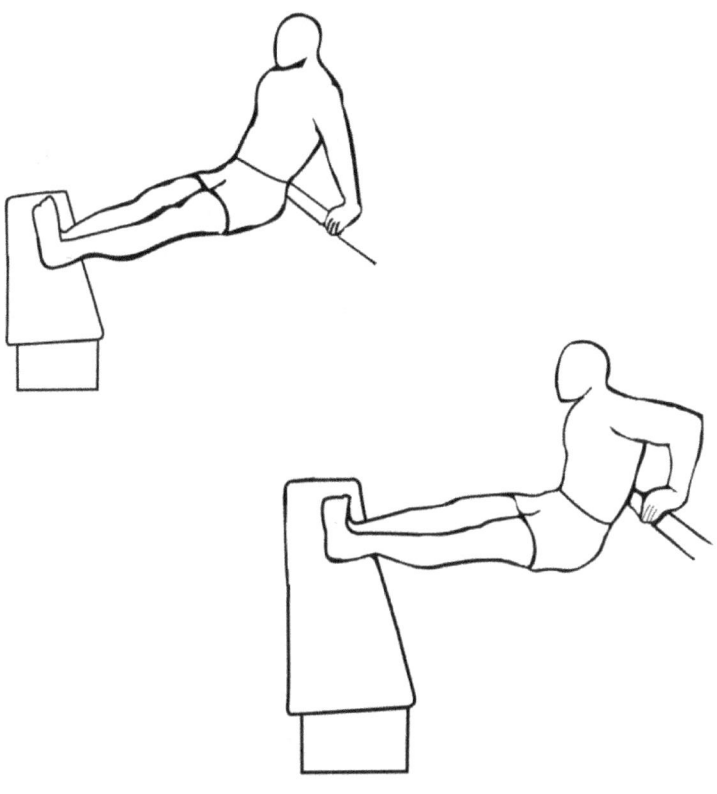

To do this exercise, position yourself at the edge of a bench by placing your hands on either side of your hips, ensuring that your fingers are positioned on the edge of the bench. Beginners can use support to balance their feet. Start by moving your buttocks off the bench little by little, bringing your feet forward. Gradually straighten your hips down in front of the bench. Now slowly lower your hips about a few inches by flexing your arms with the elbows back. After that, start pushing your body upwards while straightening your arms and keeping your shoulders even until you return to the starting position.

Leg Raises

Leg raises are fairly beginner-level exercises that strengthen the core. Start by lying down on the floor with your arms on the sides and your legs stretched out. Now start by raising your legs. At first, you might have some trouble holding your elevated legs straight up, but try to hold them as straight as possible. Your toes need to be pointed upwards.

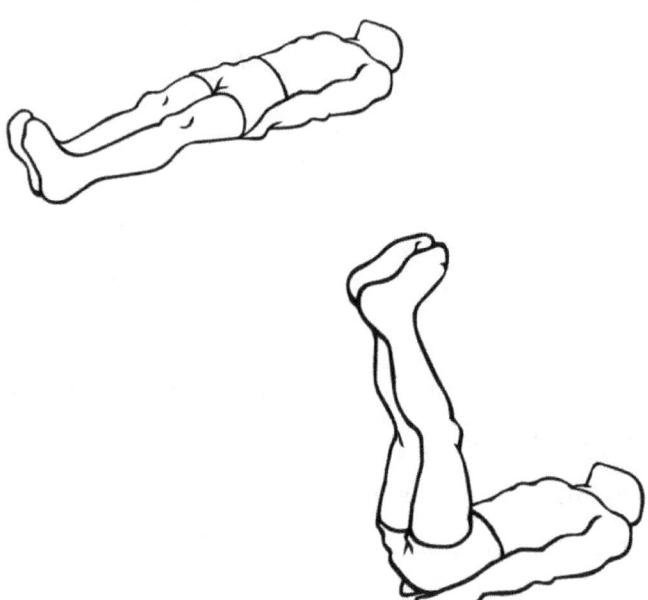

Now lower your legs back and return to starting position. Ideally, you should be shooting up to 10 reps to get the maximum benefits out of this exercise.

Street Workout for Losing Weight

Jumping Rope as a Workout

There is no question that rope jumping can have a massive effect when it comes to losing weight, gaining strength and increasing stamina. The calisthenic exercise effectively helps build more endurance, makes you stronger, and enhances your cardiovascular health. Jumping rope training also helps to condition your respiratory system, enhances blood circulation (which means more oxygen is pumped into your muscles), improves your metabolism, particularly oxygen metabolism, and helps shed excess weight.

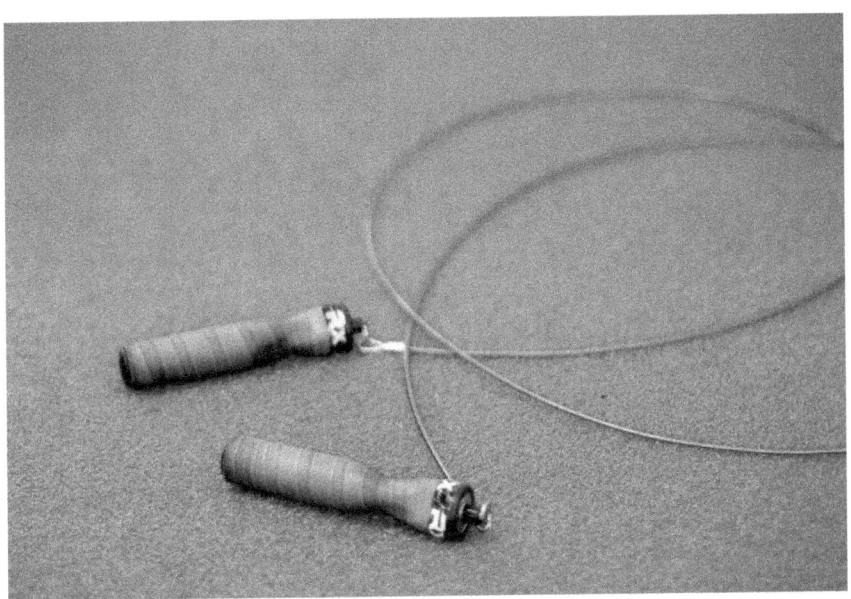

Rope jumping also tones your arms, legs and corrects your posture if you sit for long hours at work hunched in front of a computer screen. As per scientific research, it was discovered that up to 10 minutes of exercises on a jumping rope as a part of your street workout will have same effects on your metabolism, heart health and lung health, as 12 minutes of swimming, 2 sets of tennis or just running for 3 kilometers.

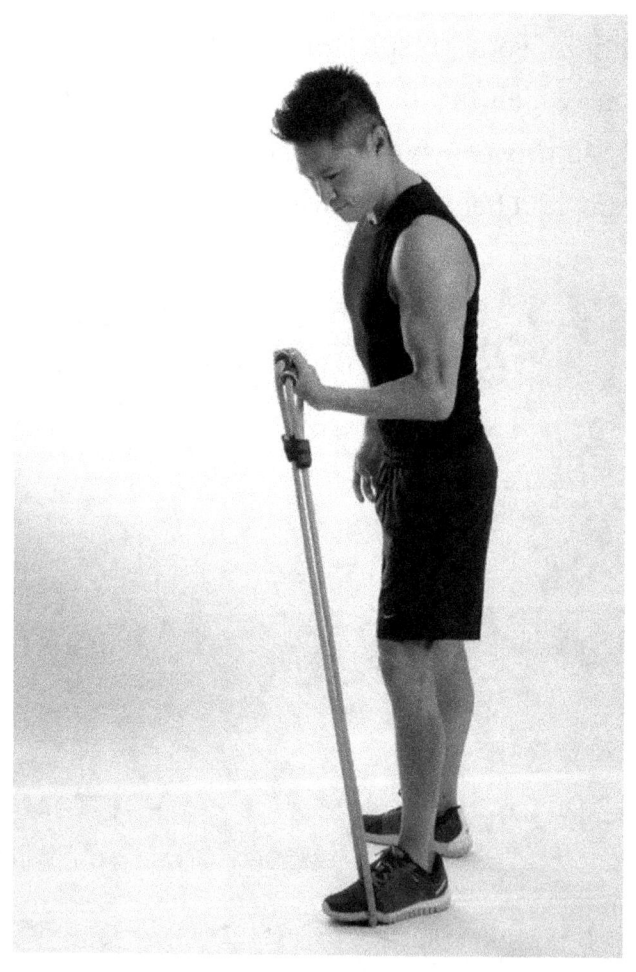

Rope jumping is without any doubts the best way of cardio training as an element of a regular calisthenic workout routine. All you need is a rope, no treadmills, no elliptical, no machine! Just a rope and you will be able to lose weight, gain stamina and improve your body's overall muscle tone. By simply jumping rope, you can burn a tremendous amount of calories compared to going swimming, taking dance classes for fitness or going out for some intense cycling.

If you're looking to burn body fat by rope jumping, the slimming effect of such exercises can only be compared to cardiovascular exercises such as running or brisk walking. If you keep on practicing for about 20 minutes every day, you will soon begin to notice beneficial changes in your overall weight. On average, a short jumping workout with proper technique will help burn about 250 to 350 calories, which is probably half the amount of calories in your dinner!

However, if your aim is not to burn fat, and you'd rather like to improve your cardiovascular health and increase your stamina, then jumping rope for around 10 to 15 minutes every day will do the trick. Nevertheless, be sure to combine rope jumping with other calisthenic exercises such as pull-ups and push-ups. And perform rope jumping exercise for no more than three times each week. Moreover, remember that the 10 to 15 timeframe is for non-stop rope jumping without any breaks in the middle of the training.

Before you grab the rope and start jumping, it is a good idea to warm up first by jump for a minute or two on the spot or performing a short jog to charge up your leg muscles. It is also a good idea to take things step-by-step, for example, don't jump for 10 minutes straight if you're doing the exercise for the first time. Jump for 2 to 3 minutes at first, and when you start to get into better shape and feel that you stamina is increasing, jump for 5 minutes straight without stopping. Jump on two feet until you master the technique, and then move on to more sophisticated variations. When you feel that strength of your legs increased enough, proceed to alternate jumps — on one leg, and then on another. You can maximize the intensity of your training by jumping in a way to skipp the rope a couple of times before landing on your feet, but that will take you a bit of time. Alternately, for increased effect you can raise your knees when jumping; you can also cross your arms and make different movements with your hands to increase intensity of the exercise.

But it is important to emphasize once more: before you do anything complicated, you have to master the basic technique! This isn't casual jumping: when you do rope jumping please ensure that your back is always straight and that your elbows are in close contact with the sides of your body. Don't jump barefoot or wearing slippers; always wear track shoes or sneakers because they will help stabilize your feet and thus minimize the chances of injury. Do not land flat-footed, your toes should touch the ground first. Exercise until it becomes difficult for you to say a sentence while jumping; if you can't and are out of breath, Give yourself a break to catch your breath back.

Buying the Right Jumping Rope

When you're looking for a jumping rope to buy, it is important to select one with sufficient length. The best way to check the length is to step at the centre of the jumpers with both your feet. If ends of the rope reach your armpits when you raise yourself a bit higher on your toes, you have rope long enough for your height.

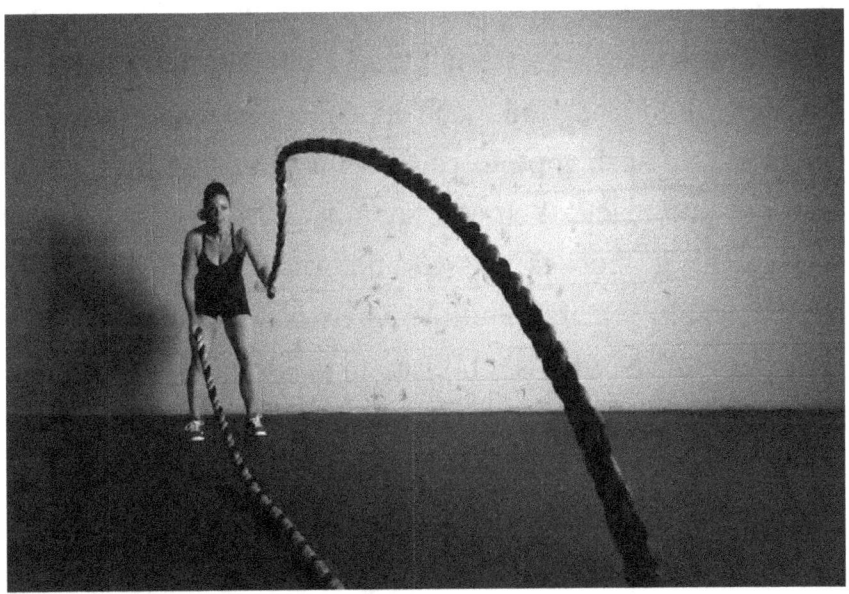

As for materials, a rubber or plastic rope will rotate quicker than a jumping rope made of soft leather or flax. But organic materials do not have that unpleasant flogging effect, which means they won't hurt you if you accidentally hit your legs or back. If you're a beginner, it's better to choose a soft-leather jumping rope. Furthermore, if you're looking to eliminate cellulite build-up or want to burn fat, choose a heavy jump rope (150-grams). You should also opt for a jump rope that has an electronic calorie counter.

In case you want to tone up your shoulders and arms, turn your attention to a jump rope with metal handles - they are heavier. Jumping ropes with built-in battery chargers have also become popular - you can charge your batteries while jumping. There are also jumping ropes for people that have low ceiling in their homes, which makes it difficult for them to rotate the rope effectively while jumping. These ropes come with laces, the materials that constitute the weight of the rope are hidden, and a cutting-edge electronic counter is installed into such rope to count your jumps as well as the rotations you made. You can say it is a virtual rope because as soon as it touches the ground, there is an automatic clicking sound, which is audible. There is an infinite choice of various products, so it is totally up to you to decide which one will work best for you.

Another important thing to mention: there are several contraindications for rope jumping that you must be aware of. If you have weak joints, problems with patella and/or intervertebral disc disease, be sure to consult your physician before performing the exercise. The same is true for people with excess weight and those suffering from hypertension or other cardiovascular conditions. Refrain from jumping if you have a migraine or a headache or if you are on a full stomach.

Advanced Level Street Workout Exercises

In this section, we will be describing advanced level street workout exercises that you should be able to master without any difficulties once you've gotten the hang of calisthenics. Here are some exercises you should try for gaining muscle mass and strength.

Push-Ups

Push-Up on Bars

Traditional push-ups are a good way to strengthen your chest, triceps, shoulders and muscles of the core body. While for some beginners doing regular push-ups on a regular basis can be a challenge, when it comes to calisthenics, you can increase your muscle tone, stamina and strength gradually by performing push-ups on bars.

To begin, hold the bars with a shoulder width grip; tilt downward until you feel your shoulders stretching comfortably.

Don't stretch your elbows out; they should be tucked close to your body. Ensure that your torso isn't too up or down; it should be perpendicular to the ground. This will be your starting position.

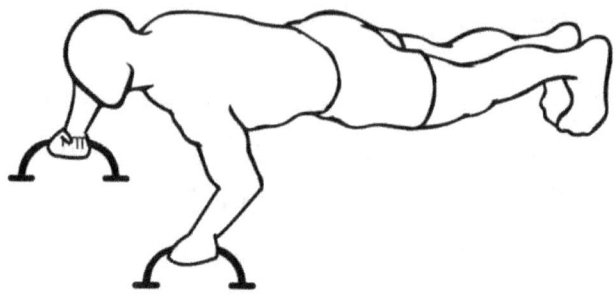

To execute the push-up movement, keep on your horizontal shoulder width firm grip on the bars, and with the grip you're holding, push your body weight up and away from the bars. For maximum effect, try to perform the push up when your chest is reaching the level of the crossbar - you are going to have to swing forward, at the top squeeze your arms. Remember that you are performing a pull-up - which means your body must not have an upwards and downwards position. Your chest and torso have to move across the bar. You can even move your legs forward so they can act as counterweights to help you keep your balance. This way performing the exercise becomes slightly complicated, which means you are going have to get used to it first.

One-Arm Push-Ups

The one-arm push-ups became immortalized in the movie Rocky; Sylvester Stallone performed the exercise with extreme focus and precision. This is a great strength building exercise; however, one-arm push-ups can be difficult for some people, yet not impossible to perform.

Go into the traditional position for push-ups, with your back straight and arms closer to your body than with regular push-ups. Try to keep your legs as far apart as you can comfortably. Doing so will help you keep your balance and to overcome twists and vibrations that will inevitably arise while you will be performing each rep. If your legs are close together, your hip joints will begin to twist, making the exercise a lot harder to complete properly. In simpler words, your body must be as straight as possible.

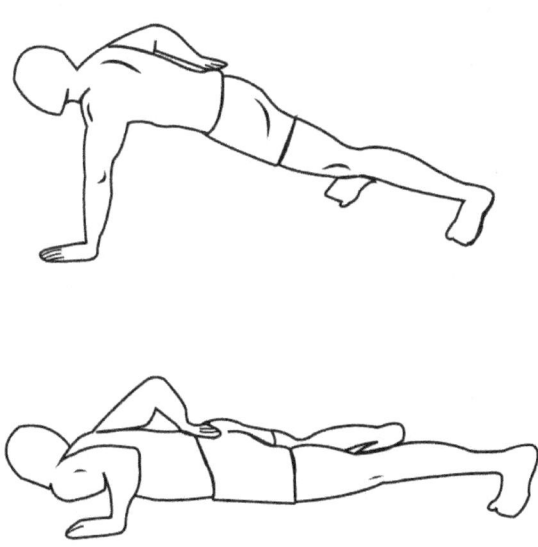

While you are maintaining this position, take away one arm from the ground and place it on your back. Slowly bend the elbow of the supporting arm and gently lower your chest.

Do not make any thrusting movements, and try to keep the elbow of the supporting arm close to your side. Lower your chest until the distance between you and ground will be only a few centimeters. Stay put for a second and then start lifting yourself back again, but do not rest or pause - keep your core, legs, and buttocks tightened during the entire set. As you strengthen your arms and lower back, you may move on to even more complicated variations such as plyometric push-ups.

One Leg Squats AKA "The Gun"

One-leg squats are an extremely difficult variation of traditional squats, which makes them even better. Well, no pain, no gain. However, even big bodybuilders who lift heavy weight when squatting have an incredibly difficult time when performing "the gun". This calisthenic exercise requires a lot of flexibility, mobility, and topnotch body balance.

This exercise doesn't fit for individuals who have weak joints, weak back muscles, and limited flexibility. Even the most experienced bodybuilder and athletes have a hard time performing one leg squats - and they do so with extreme caution.

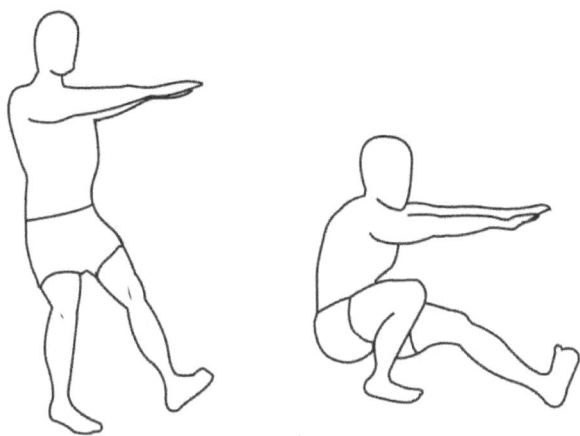

If you're up for the challenge, stand straight, lift your right or leg foot forward an make sure that your leg forms a straight line from the knee. Keep your hands forward and bend the supporting leg towards the floor. Do not bend it with the knee first; begin squatting from the hip joint and only then bend the knee. Your ankle must be as close as possible to the floor. Pause as soon as the thigh muscles at the back of your leg come close to your calf, stay put for a second and then lift yourself back to the starting position. Do not release the tension you have created in your entire body so that you can go in for the second rep right away.

Street Workouts for a Toned and Dream Body

The Human Flag

One of the most exciting exercises in street workout is the human flag. A very complex exercise with high demands to flexibility, the human flag is for people striving for pure bodily aesthetics and a powerful core. Just try to imagine a human being hanging in mid-air just like a flag, supported only by his arms holding the bar. If you're flexible enough, have strong core muscles and good balance, the task of mastering this exercise should be a bit easier for you.

Grab the pole with both hands. Keep your hands just a bit wider than the width of your shoulders. Make sure you are gripping the pole as firmly as possible. To balance your weight effectively with your lower arm, straighten it as much as you can. Use the upper arm to lift your body horizontally, keeping it strictly perpendicular to the pole. As you do this, you will feel an intense tension building in your entire body, and you need to maintain this tension. Adjust your body to stick out like a flag, you can go a bit upper or lower, or you could try bending both your feet behind the knees. Keep on practicing the movement until you can hang in the air for more than a couple of minutes or longer.

The Fro`nt Vis

Now, this is an exercise that may at first seem easy, but as you begin to perform the movement, you will wish you refrained from trying it. However, it is all in mind. Many people cannot perform this exercise simply because they do not understand the mechanics behind the movements. But even if you do know how to do it perfectly, you still need a lot of time to master the front vis.

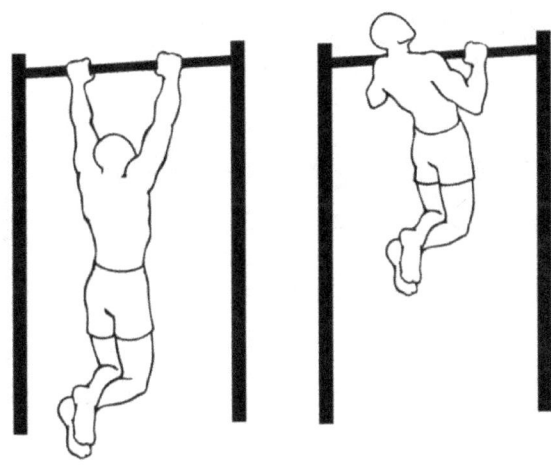

To execute the movement, you will first need to perform the active vis. Make sure that you are holding the crossbar firmly, placing your shoulders firms and moving them down. You have to maintain the tension you will feel in your entire body. With your arms straight and your elbows locked, hold the crossbar tightly and start pulling your entire body upwards, making it parallel to the floor. For a more effective movement, visualize that you are trying to pull the crossbar down to your hips. Tighten your abdominal muscles, your buttocks, and your front thigh muscles to make your body a straight line. Pull your body up, hold the position for a second or two and then lower yourself.

The Importance of Rest and Recovery

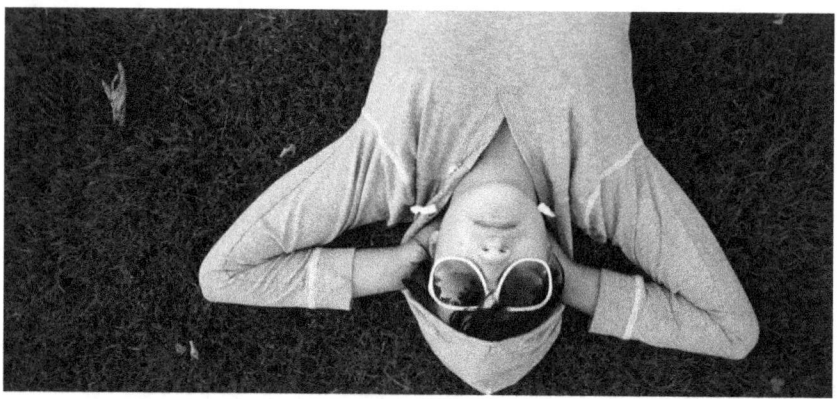

Muscle recovery time refers to the amount of time your body requires to deal with all the intensive resistance training or cardio you have been doing and heal itself after the exercise load.

You have to understand that the period of rest is in fact the very time when your training bears fruit and your muscle tone and strength increase. During the rest time or recovery period your body also replenishes the necessary energy stores your body requires to heal damaged tissues and muscle fibers. Calisthenic exercises and weightlifting both put a lot of stress on the body, maxing out its energy stores - which in scientific words is saying that your body depletes its glycogen level. Plus, there is also a fluid loss in the body as well.

Getting enough sleep and eating the right foods maximizes your body's rest and recovery. The body will start to repair all the broken muscle tissue and fibers at a faster rate, which means you will start to see more effects in a shorter span of time. Moreover, one of the core reasons why your body may shows signs of overtraining is because you aren't resting enough.

Tips on How to Gain Muscle Mass

Here are some very important tips you must know in order to maximize your gains doing calisthenic exercises. These are all simple strategies that will lead to a more toned, stronger and leaner body.

Never Stop Doing Resistance Training

Resistance training or multi-joint exercises are basically complex exercises designed to help build muscle mass. Push-ups on bars, isometric pull-ups, squatting are forms of resistance exercises that generate muscle mass.

Eat Your Proteins

When you're tearing your muscle fibers performing squats and push-ups, you need to eat the right proteins to enable your body with means to repair the torn muscle tissue. Protein sources such as boiled beef, grilled chicken, grilled fish, beans, eggs, etc. contain essential amino acids that help replace torn muscle fibers with more muscle, adding to your overall muscle tone.

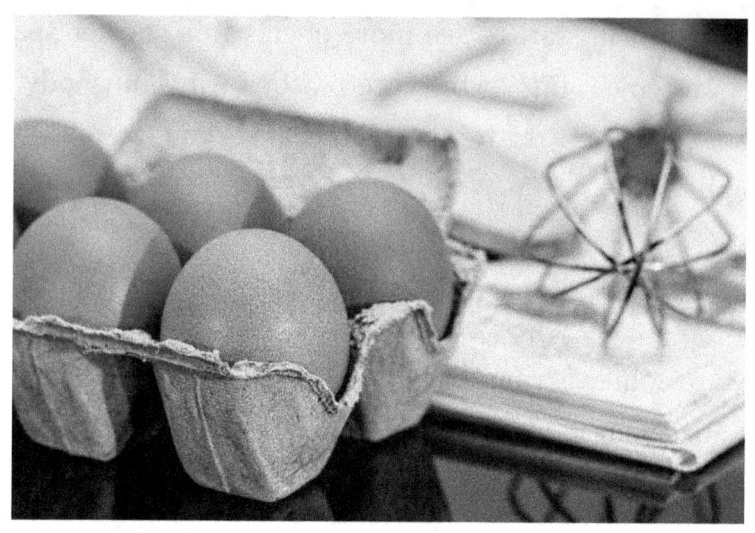

Sleep Tight and Sleep Right

Sleep for no less than 6 to 7 hours and preferably during the night hours. Sleep deprivation can become a major obstacle in gaining muscle bulk and tone. Your body repairs and heals itself just exactly during your sleep time. Thus, sleep deficit will bring to halt protein synthesis in your body.

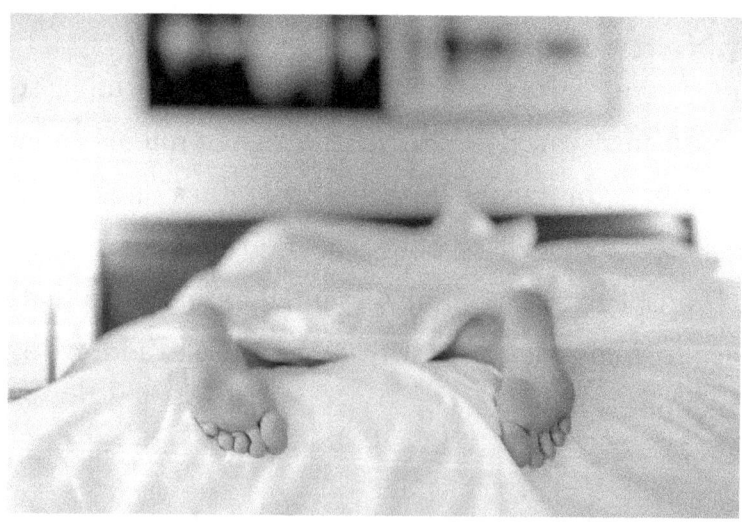

Carefully Increase your Weight

The key to increasing muscle mass is giving your body the right nutrition and at the right time. You need to be smart as to what you put inside your body. When you start your street workout, increase the load gradually; do not start with lots of repetitions.

Rest and Recovery

Understand that you will only be able to build muscle between your current and next workout session, not at the same time. That means you have to give your body a lot of rest and relaxation for it to heal. This also means eating healthy foods and watching your caloric intake. Do not skip on your protein if you're not going to work out the next day. Eat more protein and be careful not to over train your body. When it comes to calisthenics, it is recommended to schedule a workout session every other day for starters.

The Importance of a Proper Sleep Cycle for Increased Muscle Repair

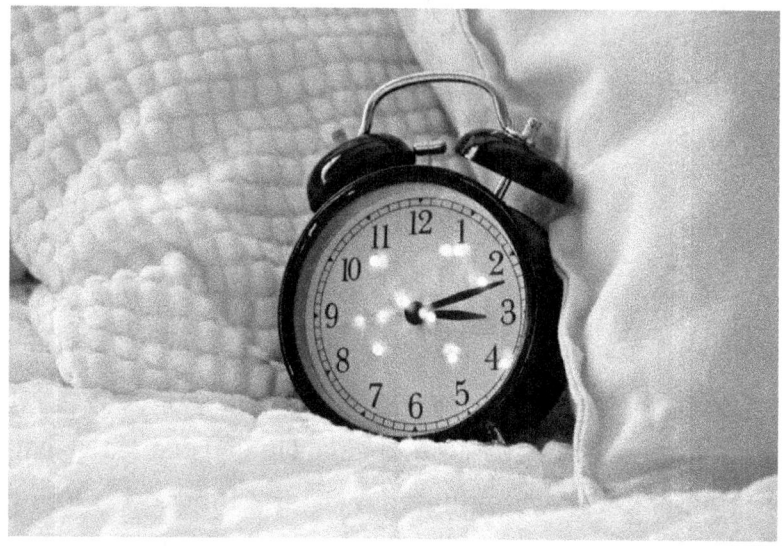

When it comes to muscle building and toning, it is a truism that you require around 7 to 8 hours of timely sleep. Sleeping on time results in more efficient muscle growth, helps your body to replenish energy stores, and repairs the brain. When you put your body under physical stress and exertion, the importance of proper sleep only increase. You can eat the healthiest foods available, you can design your workout to effectively target each body part and muscle group, and you can take all the necessary supplements; but if you are sleep deprived, you will never be able to experience the gains you want. That is because your body starts to repair all the broken and torn muscle fibers and tissues when you sleep.

Sleep deprivation causes effects that are opposite to the goals you want to achieve: you will feel moodier, you will start to gain more weight, your body will produce more stress hormones, and you will start to get hungry all the time.

There are essentially four stages of sleep:

During stage 1, you doze off, but you can wake up easily. This is where your brain cells begin to record and process all the logging movements that you have experienced throughout the day.

During stage 2, you enter into a light sleep, which is when your brain gradually begins to decrease all its activity. This is where your body calms itself down and primes for a deep sleep. Your brain starts to release growth hormones to repair torn muscle fibers and ligaments, balancing your body's metabolism.

During stage 3, your body goes into a deep sleep — it is the most vital and restorative phase of your sleep cycle. This is when your body starts to smooth your blood circulation - transferring more oxygen and blood to your muscles, repairing them with the influence of growth hormone. In addition, the brain also releases an enzyme known as prolactin, which is essential for joint repair. Overall, your body begins re-energizing itself for the morning to come.

Stage 4 is known as REM. During this phase you're in very deep sleep and start to dream or at least to experience dreaming. In the REM phase, your body rapidly increases oxygen supply to your muscles in order to break down the lactic acid build-up.

Conclusion

We're glad you've read the *Street Workout: Lose Weight and Gain Muscle Mass with Highly Effective Street Exercises* up to this last page. This information will be of great help for gaining muscle mass and finally building your dream body.

Last but not least, don't forget to leave a review for this eBook. We hope you enjoyed reading it.

www.ingramcontent.com/pod-product-compliance
Lightning Source LLC
Chambersburg PA
CBHW072114280526
45788CB00006B/2518